10-Minute Strength Training Exercises for Seniors

Stay Strong, Stay Healthy Easy Exercises for a Happier You

BY
Asterione Lyriquin

TABLE OF CONTENT

Chapter 5: Core Strength Exercises (10 minutes)

- Plank and modified plank
- Bicycle crunches

Chapter 6: Resistance Band Exercises (10 minutes)

- Using resistance bands for strength training
- Exercises for upper and lower body
- Tips for progressive overload

Chapter 7: Bodyweight Exercises (10 minutes)

- Squats, lunges, and planks without equipment
- Push-ups and tricep dips using a chair
- Leg raises and bicycle crunches

Chapter 8: Conclusion

- Summary of key takeaways

- <u>Encouragement to continue strength training</u>
- <u>Resources for further learning and support</u>

Introduction
"10-Minute Strength Training Exercises for Seniors"

Welcome to "10-Minute Strength Training Exercises for Seniors"! Our bodies naturally change as we age, which may have an impact on our balance, strength, and flexibility. Seniors can, however, lower their chance of developing chronic diseases, boost their independence, and enhance their general health and well-being with regular strength exercise.

Strength training is an essential component of healthy aging, and it's never too late to start. This book offers a senior-specific, gradually increasing intensity of strength training. 10-minute workouts are quick and efficient, and they allow you to:

- Increase energy levels and general health
- Boost muscle strength and bone density
- Improve balance and coordination
- Increase mobility and flexibility
- Lower the risk of falls and injuries

This book is perfect for seniors who:

Are inexperienced with strength training or haven't worked out in a long time; Require a mild and low-impact method; Desire to enhance their general health and well-being
Are searching for quick and effective workouts

We will walk you through a series of exercises and routines in the upcoming chapters that are specific to your needs and skill level. Always pay attention to your body, and before beginning any new fitness regimen, get advice from your healthcare provider.

Benefits of strength training for seniors

Maintaining Muscle Mass and Strength

Strength training helps seniors maintain their muscle mass and strength, which is crucial for performing daily chores and preventing deterioration.

Increased Self-Sufficiency and Movement

Regular strength training improves mobility, balance, and coordination, which reduces the risk of falls and preserves independence in older adults.

Greater Number of Years Spent in Good Health

Strength training has been shown to increase life expectancy generally and in a healthy way.

Getting Rid of Sarcopenia

Strength training can help reverse the age-related natural decline in muscular mass and strength known as sarcopenia.

An increase in bone density

Resistance training is a type of strength training activity that increases bone density and reduces the risk of fractures and osteoporosis.

Decreased Risk of Falls and Fractures

Strength training improves balance, coordination, and overall physical function, which reduces the risk of fractures and falls.

Increased vigor and strength

Strength training improves cardiovascular health and endurance, which provides seniors with increased energy and productivity to perform daily tasks.

Weight Loss and Improved Body Type

Strength training helps seniors lose weight and improve their body composition, which lowers their risk of developing chronic illnesses like diabetes and heart disease.

Enhanced Confidence and Overall Well-Being

Strength training boosts confidence and self-esteem, which benefits mental and overall wellness.

Strength training is a great way for seniors to improve their overall health and quality of life while also reaping several benefits.

Safety guidelines and precautions

Here are some safety guidelines and precautions to consider when starting a strength training program for seniors:

1. **onsult a healthcare professional**: Before starting any new exercise program, consult with a healthcare professional, especially if you have any underlying medical conditions or concerns.

2. **Warm up and cool down**: Always warm up with light cardio and stretching before strength training, and cool down with static stretches after.

3. **Start slow and progress gradually**: Begin with light weights and progress gradually to avoid injury or burnout.

4. **Focus on proper form and technique**: Prioritize proper form and technique over the number of reps or weight used.

5. **Use appropriate equipment**: Use equipment that is safe and appropriate for your fitness level, such as resistance bands or light dumbbells.

6. **Avoid overexertion**: Listen to your body and rest when needed. Avoid pushing yourself too hard, as this can lead to injury or burnout.

7. **Stay hydrated**: Drink plenty of water before, during, and after exercise to stay hydrated.

8. **Workout with a buddy or trainer**: Consider working out with a buddy or personal trainer for support and guidance.

9. **Be mindful of medications**: If you're taking medications, be aware of how they may interact with exercise and consult with your healthcare professional.

10. **Stop if you experience pain**: If you experience pain or discomfort, stop immediately and consult with a healthcare professional.

Remember, safety should always be your top priority when starting a new exercise program. By following these guidelines and precautions, you can ensure a safe and effective strength training program for seniors.

How to use this book

Welcome to "10-Minute Strength Training Exercises for Seniors"! This book is designed to help you improve your strength, flexibility, and overall health through short and effective workouts. Here's how to use this book:

1. **Start with the Introduction**: Read the introduction to learn about the benefits of strength training for seniors and how to get started.

2. **Choose Your Workout**: Select a workout from the book that suits your fitness level and goals. Workouts are labeled as "Beginner", "Intermediate", or "Advanced" to help you choose.

3. **Read the Instructions**: Read the instructions for each exercise carefully, and make sure you understand the proper form and technique before starting.

4. **Warm Up and Cool Down**: Always warm up with the provided warm-up exercises before starting your workout, and cool down with the cool-down exercises after finishing.

5. **Start with Light Weights**: Begin with light weights and gradually increase the weight as you become stronger.

6. **Focus on Proper Form:** Prioritize proper form and technique over the number of reps or weight used.

7. **Rest and Recover**: Rest for 1-2 minutes between exercises, and recover for 1-2 days between workouts.

8. **Track Your Progress**: Use the progress tracker provided to track your workouts and progress.

9. **Consult a Healthcare Professional**: If you have any concerns or questions, consult with a healthcare professional before starting any new exercise program.

By following these steps, you can get the most out of this book and achieve your strength training goals. Remember to always prioritize safety and proper form, and don't hesitate to seek help if you need it. Happy exercising!

Chapter 2:
Warm-Up and Stretching Exercises
(10 minutes)

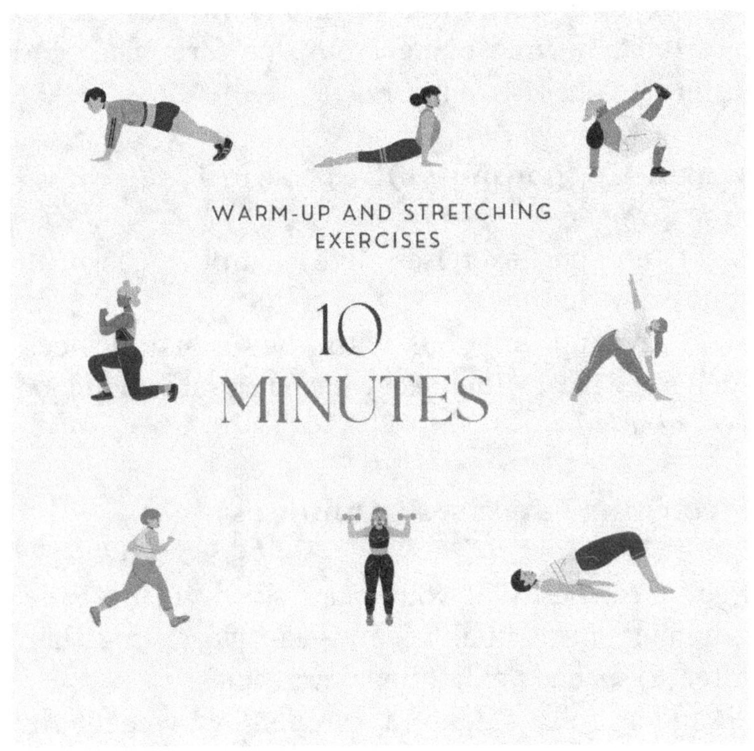

Warm-Up and Stretching Exercises (10 minutes)

It is vital to warm up and stretch your body properly before engaging in any physical activity. In the long term, this initial 10-minute investment will pay off by improving your performance and lowering your risk of injury.

Warm-Up (5 minutes)

Light aerobic exercises like jumping jacks or stationary running
Make dynamic motions with your arms and legs, such as swings; - Increase your heart rate and blood flow gradually.

Stretching Exercises (5 minutes)

Neck stretches: Tilt your head slowly to the side, bringing your shoulder and ear closer together. After 30 seconds of holding, swap sides.
Shoulder rolls: Make a circular movement by rolling your shoulders forward and backward. For thirty seconds, repeat.
Quad stretches: To maintain balance, place one hand against a wall. Maintaining your foot behind

you, bend one knee. After 30 seconds of holding,
swap legs.
To stretch your calves, stand facing a wall and place
one hand on it for balance. Keeping your heel on
the ground, take a step backwards, roughly one
foot. Lean forward and bend your front knee to
extend your calf. After 30 seconds of holding, swap
legs.

While stretching, keep in mind to breathe normally
and deeply. Avoid bouncing or exerting too much
effort on your muscles beyond what feels
comfortable.

By adding this warm-up and stretching exercise to
your daily routine, you'll decrease muscular
tension, increase your range of motion, and get
your body ready for a more efficient and injury-free
workout.

<<Gentle warm up exercises to get started>>

The following are some easy warming up exercises to get you going:

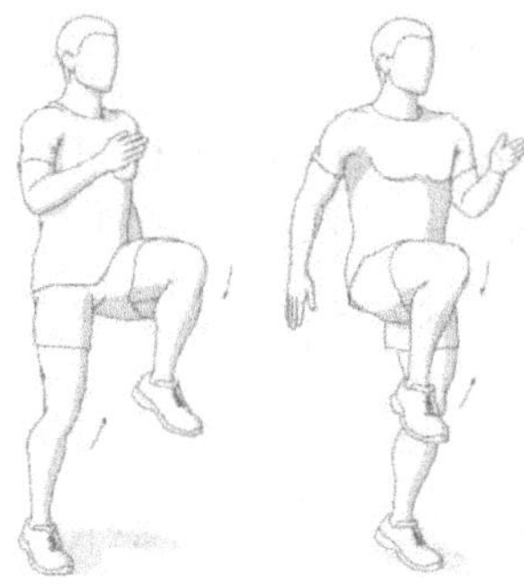

Marching in place

1. **Marching in place**: While keeping your knees close to your chest and keeping your feet hip-width apart, march in place.

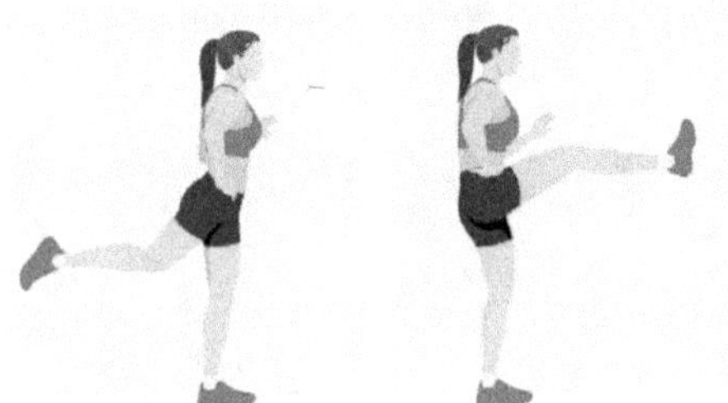

Leg Swings

2. **Leg swings**: While maintaining a hip-width distance between your feet, swing one leg forward and backward before switching to the other leg.

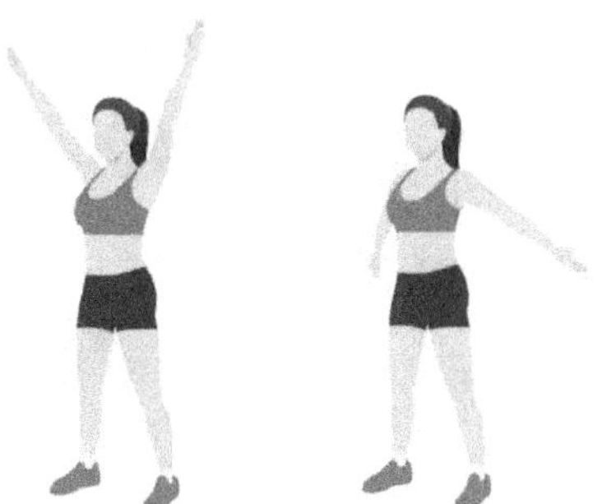

Arm circles

3. **Arm circles:** Make little circles with your hands while keeping your arms straight out to the sides.

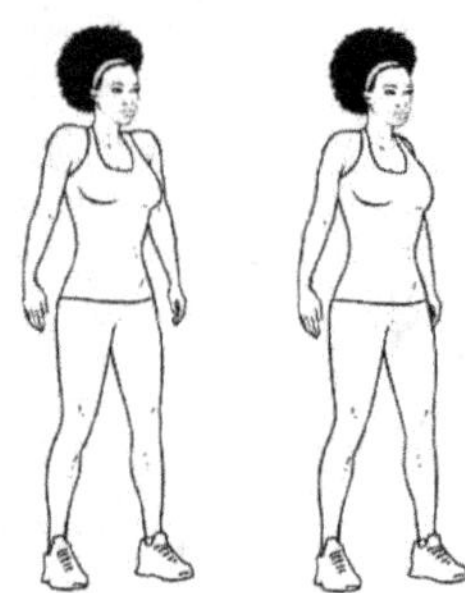

Shoulder rolls

4. **Shoulder rolls:** Make a circular movement by rolling your shoulders forward and backward.

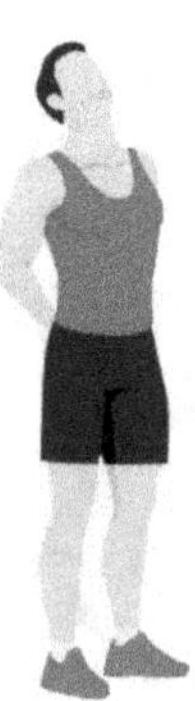

Neck stretches

5. **Neck stretches**: Gently incline your head sideways, bringing your shoulder and ear closer together. After 30 seconds of holding, swap sides.

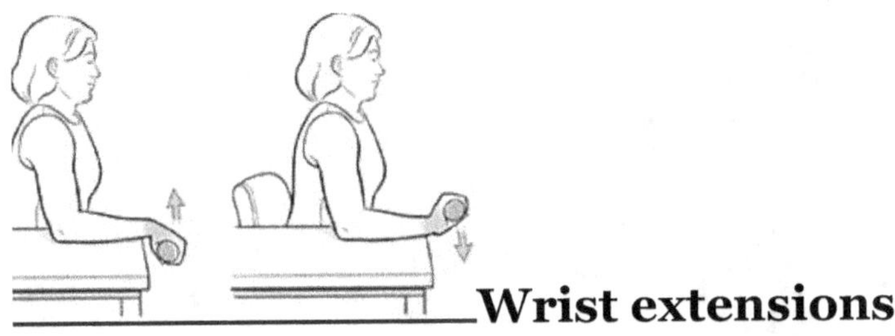

Wrist extensions

6. **Wrist extensions:** Raise and lower your hand while keeping your arm straight in front of you.

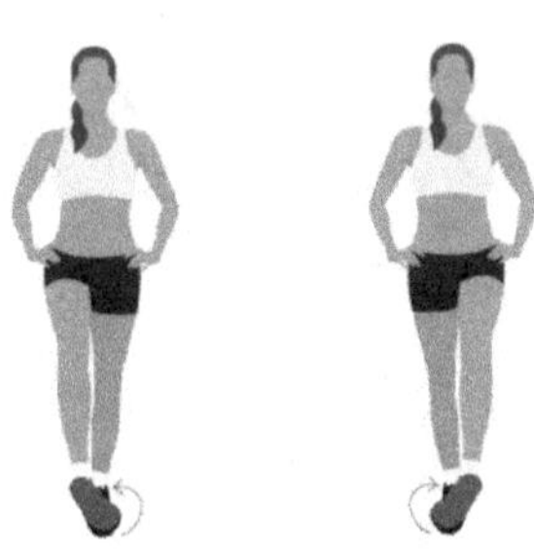

Ankle rotations

7. **Ankle rotations**: Raise your feet off the floor and make a circle with your ankles.

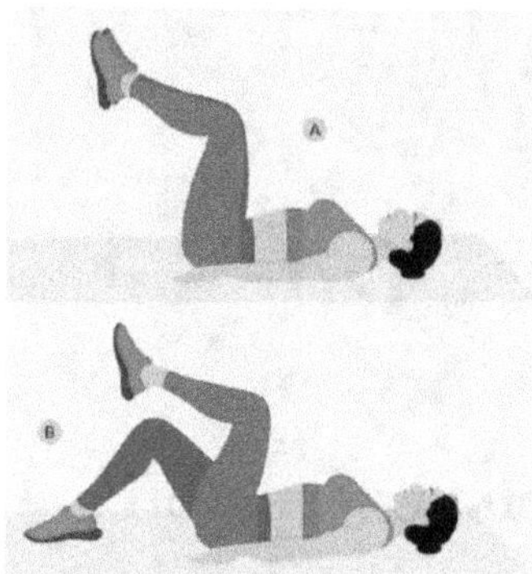

Toe taps

8. **Toe taps**: Tap your toes on the ground in front of you while standing with your feet together and one foot raised off the floor.

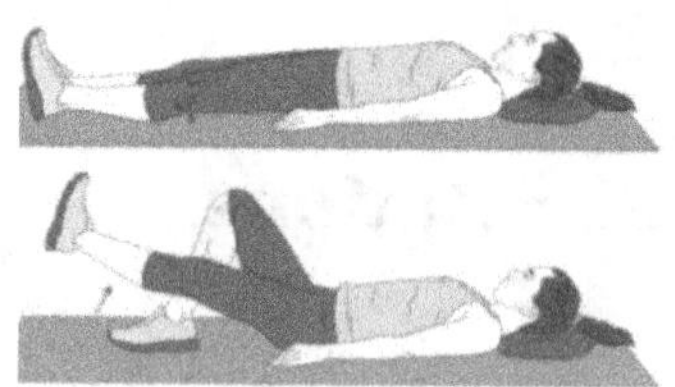

Seated leg lifts

9. **Seated leg lifts:** While sitting in a chair, raise one leg off the floor while maintaining a straight knee. After holding it for a short while, bring it back down.

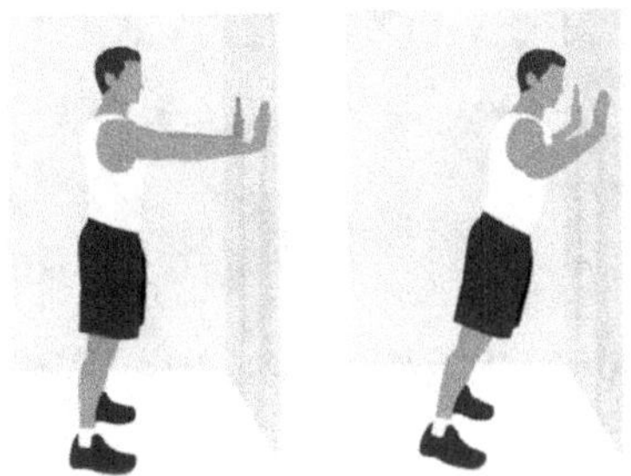

Wall push-ups

10. **Wall push-ups:** Position your hands at shoulder height on a wall while keeping your feet shoulder-width apart. Maintaining your elbows straight as you slowly lower your body toward the wall, push yourself back up to the beginning position.

As you warm up, don't forget to start off softly and gently and progressively build the intensity and time. It's also critical to pay attention to your body and to your needs, stopping if you feel pain or discomfort.

Stretching exercises to improve flexibility

The following stretches can help you become more flexible:

Upper Body

1. Chest Stretch: Plac yeour hands on the doorframe and raise your arms in a doorway. Until your chest starts to extend, lean forward. For 30 seconds, hold.
2. Shoulder Stretch: Pull your hand toward your shoulder blade with your other arm while holding one arm straight out to the side. After 30 seconds of holding, swap sides.
3. Neck Stretch: Slowly incline your head sideways, bringing your shoulder and ear closer together. After 30 seconds of holding, swap sides.

Lower Body

1. Quad Stretch: To maintain balance, place one hand against a wall. Maintaining your foot behind you, bend one knee. After 30 seconds of holding, swap legs.
2. Calf Stretch: Place one hand on the wall for balance while standing facing a wall. Keeping your heel on the ground, take a step backwards, roughly one foot. Lean forward and bend your front knee to extend your calf. After 30 seconds of holding, swap legs.
3. Hamstring Stretch: Extend your legs straight out in front of you while sitting on the floor. Reach for your toes and lean forward. Hold the position for thirty seconds.

Back and Hips

Stretch your hip flexors by kneeling on all fours. Place your foot flat on the ground in front of the opposite knee and bring one knee forward. In order to extend your hip flexor, lean forward. After 30 seconds of holding, swap sides.
2. Lower Back Stretch: Lay flat on your back with your feet flat on the floor and your knees bent. Stretch your lower back by lifting your hips off the

ground and crossing one foot over the other. After 30 seconds of holding, swap sides.

Remember

Stretching should be done with deep, natural breathing; avoid bouncing or pushing your muscles over a comfortable range of motion; hold each stretch for 30 seconds to allow for optimal muscle relaxation; and stretch frequently to show improvements in flexibility.

It's crucial to remember that flexibility exercises ought to be done painlessly and within a comfortable range. Prior to beginning any new fitness regimen, it is advisable to speak with a healthcare provider if you have any underlying medical ailments or concerns.

Chapter 3
Upper Body Strength Exercises (10 minutes)

The muscles in the arms, chest, and shoulders make up the upper body. Increasing the strength of these muscles can aid with general function, fall risk reduction, and posture. In just ten minutes, try these upper body strength exercises:

Warm-Up (1 minute)

- March in place or walk slowly
- Arm circles (forward and backward)
- Shoulder rolls (forward and backward)

Exercise 1:
Seated Arm Raises (3 sets of 10 reps)

- Sit in a chair with your feet flat on the floor
- Hold your arms straight out to the sides at shoulder height
- Raise your arms up and down

Exercise 2:
Seated Shoulder Press (3 sets of 10 reps)

- Sit in a chair with your feet flat on the floor
- Hold light weights or resistance bands at shoulder height
- Press the weights straight up over your head

Exercise 3:
Wall Push-Ups (3 sets of 10 reps)

- Stand with your feet shoulder-width apart
- Place your hands on a wall at shoulder height
- Slowly lower your body toward the wall, then push back up

Cool-Down (1 minute)

Static stretches for the shoulders, arms, and chest

As you gain strength, remember to start out slowly and progressively increase the amount of repetitions and sets. To prevent injury, it's also critical to concentrate on using correct form and technique. In the event that you feel any pain or discomfort, cease right away and get medical advice.

It is possible to modify the exercises and length according to personal fitness objectives and levels. It's crucial to speak with a medical expert before beginning a new fitness regimen.

Arm circles and shoulder rolls

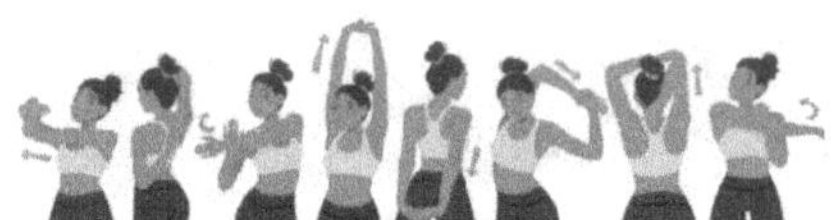

Here are some detailed instructions for arm circles and shoulder rolls:

Arm Rotations

- Raise your arms to shoulder height and hold them straight out to the sides.

- Repeat making little circles with your hands ten to fifteen times.
- Make circles in the other way after changing directions.
- Continue for three sets.

Shoulder Rolls:

1. Rotate your shoulders so they are toward your ears.
2. Roll them down and back afterwards.
3. Perform ten to fifteen repetitions.
4. Continue for three sets.

Tips:

Remain comfortable with your shoulders and arms.
1 Move smoothly and gently.
Steer clear of bouncy or jerky motions.
Inhale normally; do not hold your breath.

These exercises can ease tension and stress while also enhancing shoulder and arm range of motion and flexibility. Recall to begin cautiously and increase the amount of repetitions progressively as you gain comfort with the exercises. In the event that you feel any pain or discomfort, cease right away and get medical advice.

Push-ups and chair dips

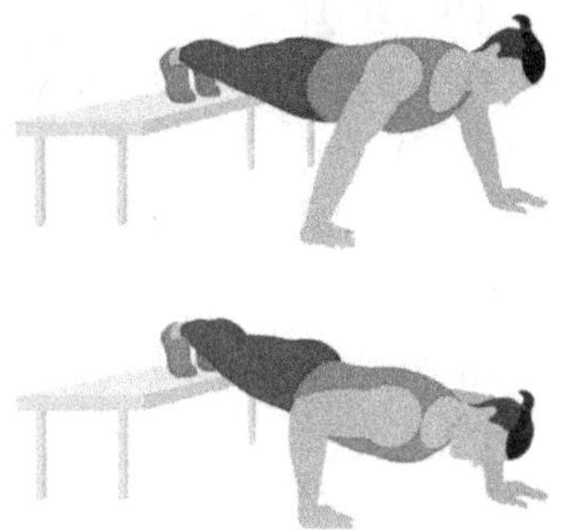

Here are some detailed instructions for push-ups and chair dips:

Push-ups

1. Begin in a plank position, placing your feet hip-width apart and your hands shoulder-width apart.
2. Bring your torso down until your chest nearly touches the floor.
3. Return to the beginning position by pushing up.

4. Perform ten to fifteen repetitions.
5. Do this three times.

Chair Dips:

1. Take a stance in front of a strong chair and hold onto the edge with your hands.
2. Bend your elbows until your arms are at a ninety-degree angle, then lower your body.
3. To get back to the beginning posture, extend your arms straight.
4. Perform ten to fifteen repetitions.
5. Do this three times.

Tips:

Maintain an engaged core and a straight body from head to heels.

- Lower yourself gradually and move with control.
- Prevent your back from arching or your hips from sagging.
- Make sure the chair you're using is stable and stable.

These workouts can help increase upper body strength and endurance, especially in the triceps, shoulders, and chest. Recall to begin cautiously and increase the amount of repetitions progressively as you gain comfort with the exercises. In the event that you feel any pain or discomfort, cease right away and get medical advice.

Bicep and tricep curls

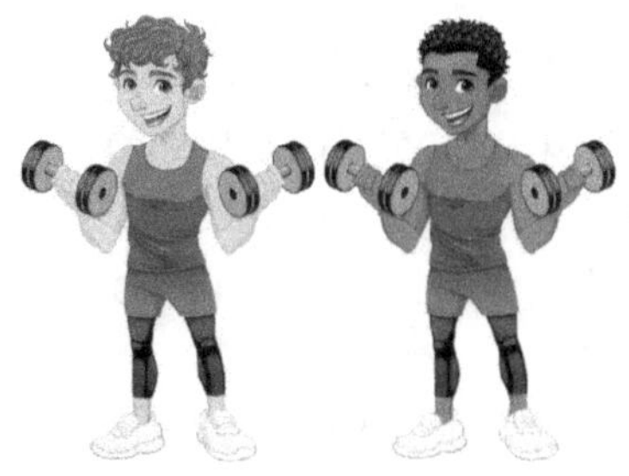

Here are some detailed instructions for bicep and tricep curls:

Bicep Curls:

1. Stand with your feet shoulder-width apart.

2. Hold light weights or resistance bands in each hand with your palms facing forward.
3. Keeping your upper arms still, bend your elbows to curl the weights up towards your shoulders.
4. Lower the weights back down to the starting position.
5. Repeat for 10-15 repetitions.
6. Repeat for 3 sets.

Curls of the Triceps:

1. Place your feet shoulder-width apart as you stand.
2. With your palm facing backward and your arm extended overhead, hold a pair of light weights or resistance bands in one hand.
3. Bend your elbow to shift the weight behind your head.
4. To get back to where you were before, extend your arm straight.
5. Continue on the opposite side.
6. Perform ten to fifteen repetitions on each side.
7. Carry out three sets of this.

Tips:

Only move your forearms; your upper arms should remain still.
Employ light weights and concentrate on deliberate motions.
Steer clear of jerking or swinging the weights.
To keep proper posture, keep your core active.

The biceps and triceps need strength and tone for daily tasks like lifting and carrying things, and these exercises can help. Recall to begin cautiously and increase the amount of repetitions progressively as you gain comfort with the exercises. In the event that you feel any pain or discomfort, cease right away and get medical advice.

Chapter 4
Lower Body Strength Exercises (10 minutes)

The lower body includes the muscles of the hips, legs, and feet. Increasing the strength of these muscles can help with mobility, fall prevention, and balance. In just ten minutes, try these lower body strength exercises:

Warm-Up (1 minute)

- Walk or march at a leisurely pace.
- Swings of the legs (forward and back)
- Clockwise and counterclockwise hip circles

Exercise 1:
Three Sets of Ten Reps of Seated Leg Lifts

Lift one leg off the ground while maintaining a straight knee - Hold for a brief period of time before lowering it back down - Repeat on the other side while seated in a chair with your feet flat on the floor.

Exercise 2:
Three sets of fifteen reps of standing calf raises

Place your feet shoulder-width apart.
Raise yourself slowly up onto your tiptoes and then descend again.

Exercise 3:
Leg Presses While Seated (3 sets of 10 reps)

Place your feet level on the floor while sitting in a chair. Then, push one leg forward while maintaining a straight knee. Hold the pose for a little while before lowering it again. Repeat on the other side.

Cool-Down (1 minute)

Stretches that are static for the feet, legs, and hips

As you gain strength, remember to start out slowly and progressively increase the amount of repetitions and sets. To prevent injury, it's also critical to concentrate on using correct form and technique. In the event that you feel any pain or discomfort, cease right away and get medical advice.

It is possible to modify the exercises and length according to personal fitness objectives and levels. It's crucial to speak with a medical expert before beginning a new fitness regimen.

Leg lifts and ankle rotations

Leg Lifts:

1. Sit in a chair with your feet flat on the floor.
2. Lift one leg off the ground, keeping your knee straight.
3. Hold for a count of 5.
4. Slowly lower your leg back down to the starting position.
5. Repeat on the other side.
6. Repeat for 10-15 repetitions on each side.
7. Repeat for 3 sets.

Ankle Rotations:

- Sit in a chair with your feet flat on the floor.
- Lift one foot off the ground and rotate your ankle in a circular motion.
- Rotate your ankle clockwise for 5-10 repetitions.
- Rotate your ankle counterclockwise for 5-10 repetitions.
- Repeat on the other side.
- Repeat for 3 sets.

Tips:

- Keep your legs straight and your feet flexed.
- Use a slow and controlled motion.
- Avoid jerky or bouncy movements.
- Keep your core engaged to maintain good posture.
- If you experience any pain or discomfort, stop immediately and consult with a healthcare professional.

The legs and ankles are vital for stability and balance, and these exercises can help increase their strength and range of motion. Recall to begin cautiously and increase the amount of repetitions progressively as you gain comfort with the exercises.

Squats and chair stands

Squats:

1. Stand with your feet shoulder-width apart.
2. Squat down gradually, maintaining a straight back and your knees behind your toes.
3. To get back up to your feet, push through your heels.
4. Perform ten to fifteen repetitions.
5. Do this three times.

Chair Stands:

1. Take a stand in front of a sturdy chair with your feet shoulder-width apart.
2. With your legs bent at a 90-degree angle and your back straight, slowly lower yourself into a sitting posture.
3. To get back up to your feet, push through your legs.
4. Perform ten to fifteen repetitions.

5. Do this three times.

Tips:

Make sure your back is straight and your core is
active.
1 Move slowly and deliberately.
Try not to let your knees go past your toes.
Step back onto your heels to stand again.
In the event that you feel any pain or discomfort,
cease right away and get medical advice.

These exercises can help increase hip and leg
strength and mobility, which is beneficial for
performing daily tasks like standing and walking.
Recall to begin cautiously and increase the amount
of repetitions progressively as you gain comfort
with the exercises.

Calf raises and toe taps

Calf Raises:

- Stand on the edge of a stair or step with your heels hanging off the edge.
- Slowly raise up onto your tiptoes, then lower back down.
- Repeat for 10-15 repetitions.
- Repeat for 3 sets.

Toe Taps:

1. Sit in a chair with your feet flat on the floor.
2. Lift one foot off the ground and tap your toes on the floor in front of you.
3. Lower your foot back down and repeat with the other foot.
4. Repeat for 10-15 repetitions on each foot.
5. Repeat for 3 sets.

Tips:

Maintain a straight kneeling position and flexed feet.
Use a slow and controlled motion.
Steer clear of bouncy or jerky motions.
To keep proper posture, keep your core active.
In the event that you feel any pain or discomfort, cease right away and get medical advice.

The calf muscles and toes are vital for stability and balance, and these workouts can help increase their strength and range of motion. Recall to begin cautiously and increase the amount of repetitions progressively as you gain comfort with the exercises.

Chapter 5
Core Strength Exercises (10 minutes)

The core muscles include the abs, obliques, and lower back. Increasing the strength of these muscles can aid in stability, balance, and posture. You can complete these 10 minute core strength exercises:

Warm-Up (1 minute)

- Walk or march at a leisurely pace.
- Swings of the legs (forward and back)
- Clockwise and counterclockwise hip circles

First exercise:
three sets of 30 seconds of planking

Begin by placing your hands shoulder-width apart in a push-up position.
To stabilize your body, use your core muscles. Hold for 30 seconds, then take a 30-second break.

Exercise 2:
Seated Russian Twists (3 sets of 10 reps)

Lean forward a little and raise your feet off the ground.
Twist your torso to the left and right, touching the ground each time. - Sit in a chair with your feet flat on the floor.

Exercise 3: Leg Raises (3 sets of 10 reps)

- Stretch your arms overhead while lying on your back.
- Raise your legs straight up toward the ceiling. Lower them back down without hitting the floor. Repeat.

Cool-Down (1 minute)

Static exercises to strengthen your core

As you gain strength, remember to start out slowly and progressively increase the amount of repetitions and sets. To prevent injury, it's also critical to concentrate on using correct form and technique. In the event that you feel any pain or discomfort, cease right away and get medical advice.

It is possible to modify the exercises and length according to personal fitness objectives and levels. It's crucial to speak with a medical expert before beginning a new fitness regimen.

Plank and modified plank

Plank:

- Start in a push-up position with your hands shoulder-width apart.
- Engage your core muscles by drawing your belly button towards your spine.
- Keep your body in a straight line from head to heels.
- Hold for 30-60 seconds.
- Rest for 30 seconds.

Modified Plank (on knees):

- Start in a plank position, but instead of having your toes on the ground, have your knees on the ground.
- Keep your body in a straight line from head to knees.
- Engage your core muscles by drawing your belly button towards your spine.
- Hold for 30-60 seconds.
- Rest for 30 seconds.

Tips:

- Remain upright and keep your shoulders away from your ears.
- Maintain a stable hip position; do not allow your hips to droop or elevate.
- To assist in supporting your body, contract your glutes.
- If necessary, take pauses and relax on your knees or in child's pose.
- In the event that you feel any pain or discomfort, cease right away and get medical advice.

If you've never done a plank before or you have any wrist or shoulder problems, the modified plank is a terrific alternative. It's also a great technique to increase your strength and stamina in preparation for a complete plank. Don't forget to concentrate on using correct form and technique; don't compromise form in order to hold the plank longer.

Bicycle crunches

Russian Twists:

1. Sit on the floor with your knees bent and feet flat.
2. Raise your feet off the ground and slant your back slightly.
3. Place a medicine ball or weight in front of your chest.
4. As you twist your torso left and right, make sure the weight is always hitting the ground next to you.
5. Repeat for 10-15 repetitions on each side.
6. Repeat for 3 sets.

Leg Raises:

1. Extend your arms upwards while lying on your back.
2. Straighten your legs and reach toward the ceiling.
3. Repeat after lowering your legs back down to the floor without touching it.
4. Perform ten to fifteen repetitions.
5. Do this three times.

Tips:

Move slowly and deliberately.
To stabilize your body, contract your core muscles.
Steer clear of jerky or momentum-based movements.
Continue to press your lower back into the earth.
In the event that you feel any pain or discomfort, cease right away and get medical advice.

Leg lifts work the lower abs, while Russian twists work the obliques. Recall to begin cautiously and increase the amount of repetitions progressively as you gain comfort with the exercises. To prevent injury, it's also critical to concentrate on using correct form and technique.

Chapter 6
Resistance Band Exercises (10 minutes)

Resistance bands are affordable, lightweight, and portable. They can be utilized to strengthen different muscle groups and offer an excellent exercise. You may complete these resistance band workouts in ten minutes or less.

Warm-Up (1 minute)

- Walk or march at a leisurely pace.
- Swings of the legs (forward and back)
- Clockwise and counterclockwise hip circles

Exercise 1:
Triple sets of 10 reps of the bicep curl

With both hands, hold the resistance band with the palms facing forward.
Curl your arms upward while maintaining the same posture for your upper arms.
Return to the beginning position by lowering your arms.

Exercise 2:
Triple Sets of Ten Reps for Tricep Extension

Lower your hand behind your head while maintaining the motion of your upper arm. - Hold the resistance band in one hand with your arm extended overhead.
Return your hand to its initial position.

Exercise 3:
Triple Set Chest Press (10 Reps)

- Raise both hands to shoulder height;
- Press the resistance band forward to completely extend your arms;
- Lower your arms back to the starting position.

Exercise 4:
Rotating Shoulders (3 sets of 10 repetitions)

Raise your arm straight and rotate your shoulder in a circular motion while holding the resistance band in one hand at shoulder height.
Repeat on the opposite side.

Cool-Down (1 minute)

Arm and shoulder stretches that are static

Remember to start slowly and gradually increase the number of reps and sets as you become more comfortable with the exercises. To prevent injury, it's also critical to concentrate on using correct form and technique. In the event that you feel any pain or discomfort, cease right away and get medical advice.

It is possible to modify the exercises and length according to personal fitness objectives and levels. It's crucial to speak with a medical expert before beginning a new fitness regimen.

Using resistance bands for strength training

Resistance bands are a great tool for strength training! They provide an affordable, adaptable, and portable form of exercise. The following are some advantages and pointers for strength training with resistance bands:

Benefits:

Compared to typical weights or gym equipment, their portability and lightweight make them easier to carry with you on the move. They are also less expensive. You may use them to work out different muscle areas, such as the arms, legs, chest, back, and shoulders.

- Maintain constant tension throughout the range of motion to enhance flexibility and strength.
- Low-impact, which means that joints are less strained than with large weights or high-impact workouts

Tips:

- Select the appropriate resistance level based on your goals and level of fitness.

- Start with gentler movements and then increase speed as you grow more comfortable.
- Use good form and technique to avoid injury.
- Use resistance bands in conjunction with other exercises, such as bodyweight exercises or cardio, for a comprehensive workout.
- Incorporate a range of exercises to target different muscle groups.
- To boost the intensity and versatility of your workout, think about incorporating handles or anchors.

Several well-liked resistance band exercises consist of:

- Shoulder rotations
- Leg curls and extensions
- Bicep curls
- Tricep extensions
- Chest presses
- Rows

Do not forget to seek medical advice before to beginning any new fitness regimen.

Exercises for upper and lower body

Upper Body:

- Bicep curl: With your palms pointing forward, hold the band in both hands. Keep your upper arms motionless as you curl them up.
- Tricep Extension: Raise your arm overhead while holding the band in one hand. Raise your hand back up after lowering it behind your head.
- Chest Press: Raise the band to shoulder height with both hands. Fully extend your arms by pressing the band forward.
- Shoulder Rotation: Raise one hand to shoulder height and hold the band there. With your arm straight, rotate your shoulder in a circular motion.
- Lateral Raise: Raise the band to shoulder level with both hands. Keep your arms straight as you extend them out to the sides.

Lower Body:

1. Leg Curl: Fasten the band to something sturdy. With both hands on the band, twist your legs up while maintaining a bent knee.
2. Leg Extension: Secure the band to something sturdy. Maintain a straight posture with your legs while holding the band with both hands.
3. Hip Abduction: Raise the band to your hip level with both hands. Stretch your legs apart without bending them.
4. Hip Adduction: At hip height, hold the band with both hands. Keep your legs straight as you bring them together.
5. Calf Raise: Fix the band to something sturdy. Raise your heels while maintaining a straight knee while grasping the band with both hands.

Remember to start with lighter resistance and gradually increase as you become stronger. To prevent injury, it's also critical to concentrate on using correct form and technique.

Tips for progressive overload

Progressive overload is a training principle that involves gradually increasing the intensity of your workouts to build strength and muscle. Some advice for progressive overload is as follows:

1. Increase the weight: To put more strain on your muscles, gradually raise the weight you lift over time.
2. Increase the reps: To build muscle endurance, gradually increase the amount of repetitions you perform.
3. improve the sets: To improve overall volume, incorporate extra sets into your exercise regimen.
4. Shorten rest periods: To raise intensity, gradually shorten the intervals between sets and workouts.
5. Increase frequency: To push your muscles more frequently, up the frequency of your workouts.

6. Switch up your workouts: Gradually move up to harder workouts, including going from machine-based to free-weight exercises.
7. Expand range of motion: To give your muscles a greater challenge, expand the range of motion during your workouts.
8. Extend time under tension: During exercises, extend the amount of time your muscles are under tension.
9. Put an emphasis on progressive overload in little increments: Make it a habit to progressively increase weight, reps, or sets by tiny amounts (2.5–5 pounds, 1-2 reps, or 1 set).
10. Be Consistent: Training frequently and creating the habit of progressive overloading are important aspects of progressive overloading.

Remember, progressive overload should be done gradually and consistently to avoid injury or burnout. It's critical to pay attention to your body and modify your exercise regimen as necessary.

Chapter 7
Bodyweight Exercises (10 minutes)

Bodyweight exercises are a great way to improve strength and flexibility without needing any equipment. You can complete the following bodyweight exercises in ten minutes or less:

Warm-Up (1 minute)

Walk or march at a leisurely pace.
Swings of the legs (forward and back)
Clockwise and counterclockwise hip circles

Exercise 1
Three sets of ten push-ups

Place your hands shoulder-width apart and begin in the plank posture.
Push yourself back up to the beginning posture after lowering your body until your chest almost touches the ground.

Exercise 2
 Squats (3 sets of 10 reps)

Place your feet shoulder-width apart as you stand.
Keep your back straight as you lower yourself into a
squat.
Return to the starting position by pushing up.

Exercise 3
Lunges (3 sets of 10 reps)

Maintaining a straight back, lower your body into a
lunge while standing with your feet together. Push
yourself back up to the starting position and repeat
with the other leg.

Exercise 4
Plank Hold (3 sets, 30-second hold)

Place your hands shoulder-width apart to begin in
the plank position.
Hold this position for 30 seconds while using your
core muscles.

Cool-Down (1 minute)

Arm, leg, and back stretches that are static

Remember to start slowly and gradually increase the number of reps and sets as you become more comfortable with the exercises. To prevent injury, it's also critical to concentrate on using correct form and technique. In the event that you feel any pain or discomfort, cease right away and get medical advice.

Squats, lunges, and planks without equipment

Squats:

Place your feet shoulder-width apart.
Squat down, maintaining a straight back and your knees behind your toes.
Push yourself back up to the starting position.
Pay attention to maintaining your core engaged and your weight in your heels.

Lunges

Keep your back straight and your front knee behind your toes as you lower yourself into a lunge. Push yourself back up to the starting position and repeat with the other leg. Pay attention to maintaining your core engaged and your weight in your front heel. Stand with your feet together.

Planks:

Hold yourself up straight from head to heels, rather than lowering your body.
Begin in the push-up posture with your hands shoulder-width apart.
Focus on maintaining your body straight and your core engaged.
Use your core muscles to support your body.
Hold for as long as you can, aiming for at least 30 seconds.

Remember to:

Increase the amount of repetitions and sets gradually as you get more accustomed to the workouts.
Pay attention to correct form and technique to prevent injuries; pay attention to your body and take breaks when necessary; seek medical advice if you have any concerns or injuries.

Push-ups and tricep dips using a chair

Push-ups:

- Take a stance in front of a stable chair and hold onto the edge with your hands.
- Drop your torso until your arms are positioned 90 degrees apart.
- Return to the beginning position by pushing up.
- Continue for the required number of repetitions.

Tricep dips:

- Take a stance in front of a stable chair and hold onto the edge with your hands.
- Bend your elbows until your arms are at a 90-degree angle in order to lower your body.
- To get back to the beginning posture, extend your arms straight.
- Continue for the required number of repetitions.

Tips:

Verify that the chair is stable and won't move as you perform the exercise.
Maintain a straight posture and contract your core muscles.
Slowly descend and maintain control over your motions.
As your strength increases, progressively increase the number of reps and sets you begin with.

If you're just starting out or have mobility limitations, using a chair to perform push-ups and tricep dips is a terrific method to adapt the workouts and make them more accessible. To prevent injuries, always put good form and technique first.

Leg raises and bicycle crunches

Leg raises and bicycle crunches are two effective exercises for strengthening your core muscles. Here's how to carry them out:

Leg Raises:

1. Lay flat on your back with your legs straight and your arms outstretched overhead.
2. Straighten your legs as you raise them off the ground.
3. Lift your legs to the ceiling and then return them to the floor without making contact with it.
4. Continue for the required number of repetitions.

Bicycle Crunches:

1. Assume a prone position, placing your hands behind your head and bending your knees 90 degrees.
2. Bend your knees in alternate directions toward your chest, as you're pedaling a bike.
3. Concentrate on using your abdominal muscles to raise your shoulders off the floor.
4. Continue for the required number of repetitions.

Tips:

As you get more accustomed to the exercises, start with gentler movements and then pick up the pace.
Rather than depending solely on momentum, concentrate on using your core muscles to raise your shoulders and legs.
Steer clear of hunching over or elevating your head and shoulders with your hands.
Recall to inhale normally and not to hold your breath.

To prevent injuries, always put good form and technique first. Before beginning any new workout regimen, it's a good idea to speak with a healthcare provider or fitness specialist if you have any underlying medical ailments or concerns.

Conclusion

Congratulations on completing the 10-Minute Strength Training Exercises for Seniors program! You've made a big improvement to your general health and wellbeing by including these activities into your everyday regimen.

Remember, strength training is an important part of maintaining independence and quality of life as we age. Gaining strength and endurance will help you accomplish everyday chores more easily, lower your chance of getting sick or injured, and improve your general physical and mental well-being.

Here are some last pointers to bear in mind:

- Include strength training in your daily routine to make it a habit; - Increase the intensity and duration of your workouts gradually; - Pay attention to your body and take breaks when necessary; - Drink plenty of water and eat a healthy diet; - Think about working with a personal trainer or fitness coach to create a personalized strength training program.

Thank you for choosing the 10-Minute Strength Training Exercises for Seniors program. We really hope you've enjoyed and found it useful. Always put your health and wellbeing first, and don't stop strength training!

Summary of key takeaways

Key learnings from the "10-Minute Strength Training Exercises for Seniors" program are outlined below:

For seniors to retain their independence and quality of life, strength training is essential. Start with short, easy workouts (10 minutes), then progressively increase the time and intensity. Put more emphasis on perfect form and technique than on the number of reps and sets.
Make strength training a habit by incorporating it into your daily routine.- Employ bodyweight, resistance bands, or light weights for exercises.- Give priority to exercises that improve balance, flexibility, and core strength.- Pay attention to your body and take breaks when necessary.-Consider working with a personal trainer or fitness coach for individualized guidance.

Recall that growth, not perfection, is the aim! You can raise the quality of your life by implementing these important lessons into your strength training regimen.

Encouragement to continue strength training

Thank you for starting the journey to a better, more confident version of yourself! Every repetition, every set, and every workout is a win in the road that is strength training. Recall your starting point and your progress. If you skip a day or two, don't be too hard on yourself; just get back on track and carry on.

With every day that goes by, you continue to gain confidence, strength, and endurance. Your diligence and commitment will be rewarded, and the outcomes will be worthwhile. Maintain your momentum and don't forget to acknowledge and appreciate your little victories along the way.

You are capable of this! Continue pushing, lifting, and shining!

Recall that strength training focuses on resilience and mental toughness in addition to physical strength. Both your body and mind are getting stronger. Continue forth and have faith in your ability to do amazing things!

Resources for further learning and support

The following resources can help you learn more and provide support

1. Manager: Your boss is one of the greatest people to talk to about your personal development goals and get advice and comments on how to advance both professionally and personally.
2. Coworkers: Coworkers can offer performance reviews and guidance on achieving career goals. Their tactics and

methods of making decisions can also teach you.

3. Mentor: A mentor may help you succeed both personally and professionally by offering counsel, direction, and support. It is possible to integrate good habits into your own by paying attention to them and taking their recommendations.

4. Both formal and informal training: Learning and personal growth can be enhanced by training initiatives. Formal training may be offered by your workplace or by outside organizations. To develop your skills, you can also enroll in online classes.

5. Team meetings: These might provide you and your teammates the chance to learn something new together. To find a solution, you can talk about common issues and exchange ideas.

6. Seminars: Attending local seminars might advance one's professional or personal development. You can use the knowledge from these workshops in both your personal and professional life.

7. Workshops: These gather professionals with specialized knowledge in one location. Attendees must actively participate in these

workshops. Gaining practical experience can help you develop new abilities.

8. Volunteering: Participating in volunteer work provides an opportunity to develop your communication and practical abilities.

9. Conducting research online: The Internet is a useful tool for learning and staying current.

10. Books: You can get better by reading books that you find interesting and that are related to your professional and personal development.